The Definitive Mediterranean Dessert Collection

Get Ready to Make Healthy and Affordable Dessert and Boost Your Metabolism

Lexi Robertson

Table of contents

Black Forest

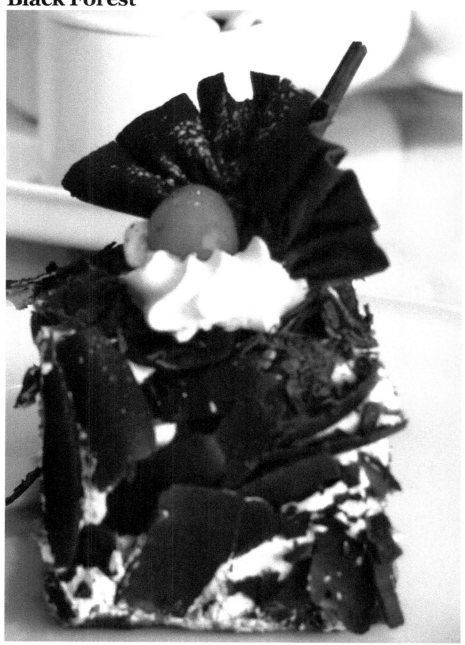

Difficulty Level: 2/5

Preparation time: 5 minutes

Cooking time: 23 minutes

Servings: 8-10

 Ingredients:

1 box of chocolate cake mix; use 2 cups

1 cup skim milk

2 eggs

2 cups of double cream (heavy whipping cream)

1 teaspoon icing sugar (powdered sugar)

1 teaspoon vanilla extract

¼ cup unsweetened cocoa powder unsweetened cocoa powder

24 jar maraschino cherries (12 cut in half and 12 whole to decorate)

1 cup cherries juice

½ cup grated chocolate (chocolate shavings)

Oil spray

Directions:

In a bowl, add the cake mix, milk and eggs. Combine well.

Preheat the skillet at medium-high temperature for 3 minutes; Remove the pan from the pot for 1 minute and lightly spray the oil spray. Pour the cake mixture into the pan, cover with the valve closed, lower the temperature to low and cook for approximately 20-23 minutes, or until a knife is inserted, it comes out clean.

In the other bowl, add the double cream, sugar and vanilla extract. Beat until it thickens. Divide this cream into two equal parts. Mix one of the parts with the cocoa powder, and the other with the cherries in halves.

7

Slice the chocolate cake in two layers and drill holes in each with the help of a knife. Pour the cherry juice into both layers.

Spread the cream mixture with cherries over the bottom layer. Place the second layer on top and cover with the cream and cocoa mixture. Garnish with whole cherries, grated chocolate and cocoa powder. It can be served immediately or refrigerated for 30 minutes.

Nutrition:

Calories: 539

Carbohydrates: 54g

Fat: 33g

Protein: 8g

Sugar: 29g

Cholesterol: 115mg

Ripe Banana Pudding
Difficulty Level: 2/5

Preparation time: 5 minutes

Cooking time: 25 minutes

Servings: 8

Ingredients:

1 pound (½ kg) of white / square white bread, in thick slices

1 can of condensed milk (14 oz/396 ml)

1 can of evaporated milk (12 oz/354 ml)

1 cup coconut milk

3 beaten eggs

½ cup Marsala wine (optional)

2 ripe bananas chopped into small pieces

½ cup pecan nuts (optional)

1 teaspoon vanilla extract

1 teaspoon ground cinnamon

½ teaspoon nutmeg powder

1 teaspoon whole wheat flour (optional)

Oil spray

Directions:

Chop the bread into medium cubes. Place it in the bowl, and pour half of the condensed milk, half of the evaporated milk and half of the coconut milk. Stir well.

Add the beaten eggs, wine, bananas, nuts, vanilla extract, cinnamon and nutmeg. Combine and let the bread absorb the mixture for about 15 minutes.

Meanwhile, in the pot, mix the remaining 3 milks (evaporated, condensed and coconut), and cook for 8 minutes at medium temperature, or until they begin to thicken. Stir occasionally. If you need thickness, add whole wheat flour.

Preheat the skillet over medium heat for 2 minutes, sprinkle oil spray, and add the bread mixture.

Reduce the temperature to low, cover and cook for 18 minutes.

Remove the pan from the pot and let stand for about 5 minutes.

Serve and pour a little of the milk mixture in each serving.

Nutrition:

Calories: 288

Carbohydrates: 47g

Fat: 10g

Protein: 4g

Sugar: 34g

Cholesterol: 6.5mg

Picositos Brownies

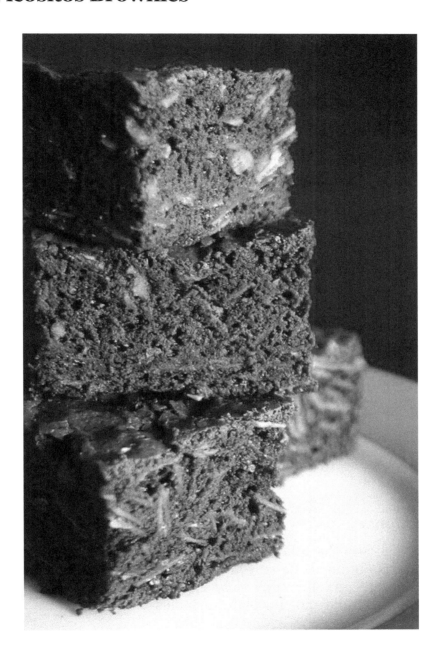

Difficulty Level: 2/5

Preparation time: 5 minutes

Cooking time: 15 minutes;

Servings: 8

Ingredients:

3 cups brownies mix

2 eggs

1/3 cup of milk

½ teaspoon cayenne pepper

1 teaspoon cinnamon

1 teaspoon vanilla extract

¼ cup chocolate sprinkles

Liquid candy to taste (decoration)

Chocolate sauce to taste (decoration)

Oil spray

Directions:

In a bowl, stir the following ingredients until a homogeneous mixture is obtained. Be sure to add them little by little, in the same order: mix for brownies, eggs, milk, cayenne pepper, cinnamon, vanilla and chocolate sprinkles.

Preheat the skillet at medium-high temperature for 2 and a half minutes. Cover the pot with the spray oil and reduce the temperature to low. Make sure the oil does not start to burn.

Add the previous mixture immediately, cover with the valve closed and cook for 15 minutes. Turn off the pot, remove the pan from the burner and let it sit for 3 minutes. Carefully invert the brownies on the Bamboo Cutting Board, slice it and serve with caramel or chocolate sauce.

Nutrition:

Calories: 539

Carbohydrates: 54g

Fat: 33g

Protein: 8g

Sugar: 29g

Cholesterol: 115mg

Fruit Crepes

Difficulty Level: 2/5

Preparation time: 5 minutes

Cooking time: 15 minutes

Servings: 4

Ingredients:

Crepes:

1 cup wheat flour

2 eggs

1¼ cups of milk

1 teaspoon vanilla extract

2 tablespoons melted butter

a pinch of salt

Powdered sugar to taste (powdered sugar)

Olive oil spray

Filling

2 cups of strawberries, sliced

½ cup sour cream

¼ cup brown sugar

1 teaspoon vanilla extract

Directions:

In a bowl, combine the flour and eggs. Add the milk gradually. Then add the vanilla extract, butter, salt and icing sugar. Beat well until you get a homogeneous mixture.

In the other bowl, combine the filling ingredients well with the help of the Spatula.

Preheat the skillet at medium-high temperature for about 2 and a half minutes and immediately lower the temperature to low. Cover the pan with olive oil spray.

With the help of the ladle, add approximately 1/8 cup of the mixture in the pan. Tilt the pan slightly to allow the mixture to spread evenly across the surface.

Cook the crepes for 40 to 45 seconds per side, or until lightly browned. Use the Silicone Spatula to flip them.

Repeat steps 4 and 5 with the remaining mixture. Add more spray oil, if necessary.

Fill the crepes and serve with syrup.

Nutrition:

Calories: 101

Carbohydrates: 17g

Fat: 1.4g

Protein: 6g

Sugar: 5g

Cholesterol: 43.4mg

Vanilla Cake

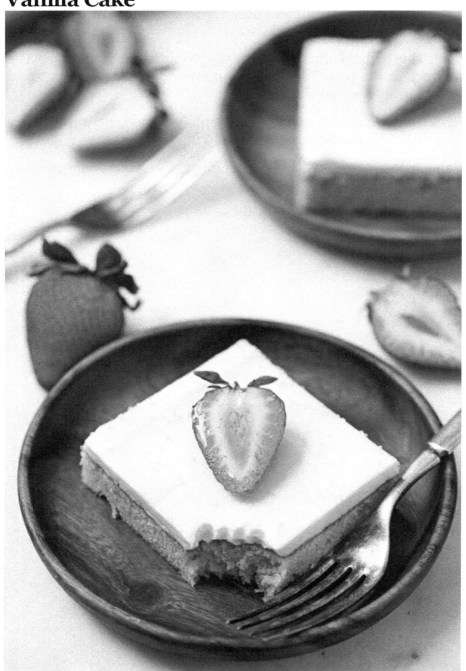

Difficulty Level: 2/5

Preparation time: 5 minutes

Cooking time: 23 minutes

Servings: 12

Ingredients:

 Flan*:*

1 cup of condensed milk

1 cup evaporated milk

3 eggs

1 teaspoon vanilla extract

Cake*:*

2 cups of chocolate cake mix

2 eggs

¾ cup of nonfat milk

Oil spray

Directions:

Flan:

Blend condensed milk, evaporated milk, 3 eggs and vanilla extract for 2 minutes. Reserve this mix

Cake:

In the bowl, combine the cake mix, eggs and milk with the help of the Balloon Whisk. Reserve this preparation.

Preheat the pan at medium-high temperature for 3 minutes; Remove the pan from the stove for 1 minute and lightly spray the spray oil all over the surface - including the walls of the pan.

Add the cake mixture to the pan. With the help of a spoon, pour the flan mixture evenly. Put the pan back on the pot, reduce the temperature to low, cover with the valve closed and cook for 23 minutes.

Let the pan rest for a few minutes. Turn it carefully, so that the cake falls on a plate or flat surface. Slice it and serve.

Nutrition:

Calories: 84.62

Carbohydrates: 1g

Fat: 7.02g

Protein: 3.71g

Sugar: 0.64g

Cholesterol: 97.43mg

Vanilla Pastry Cream
Difficulty Level: 2/5

Preparation time: 5 minutes

Cooking time: 5 minutes

Servings: 4

Ingredients:

2 cups low fat milk

2 lightly beaten eggs

¼ cup sugar

¼ teaspoon salt

½ teaspoon of vanilla

Nutmeg

1 cup of water

Directions:

Combine milk, eggs, sugar, salt and vanilla and pour into individual cups for custard. Sprinkle with nutmeg.

Cover each cup firmly with the foil. Pour the water into the pot. Position the cups on the rack of the pot.

Close and secure the lid. Place the pressure regulator on the vent tube and cook 5 minutes once the pressure regulator begins to rock slowly.

Cool the pot quickly. Let the cream cool well in the refrigerator.

Nutrition:

Calories: 137

Small Pumpkin Pastry Cream
Difficulty Level: 2/5

Preparation time: 5 minutes

Cooking time: 10 minutes

Servings: 8

Ingredients:

1 can of 16 ounces of prepared pumpkin

1 14-ounce can sweetened condensed milk

3 beaten eggs

1 teaspoon finely chopped polished ginger (optional)

1 teaspoon ground cinnamon

¼ teaspoon ground cloves

1 cup of water

Directions:

Mix the pumpkin, milk, eggs, cinnamon, ginger and cloves. Pour into individual cups for custard.

Cover each cup firmly with the foil. Pour the water into the pot. Position the cups on the rack of the pot. Close and secure the lid.

Place the pressure regulator on the vent tube and cook 10 minutes once the pressure regulator begins to rock slowly. Cool the pot quickly. Let the cream cool well in the refrigerator. If desired, serve with whipped cream.

Nutrition:

Calories: 207

Tapioca Pudding

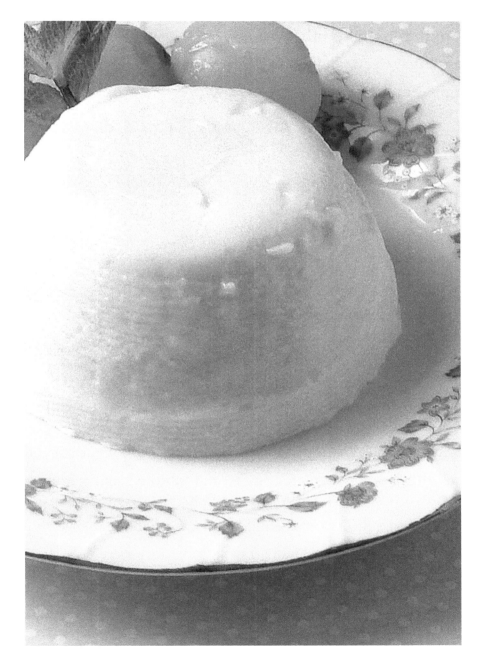

Difficulty Level: 2/5

Preparation time: 5 minutes

Cooking time: 20 minutes

Servings: 6

Ingredients:

2 cups low fat milk

2 tablespoons quick-cooking tapioca

2 lightly beaten eggs

⅓ cup of sugar

½ teaspoon of vanilla

1 cup of water

Directions:

Heat the milk and tapioca. Remove from heat and let stand 15 minutes.

Combine eggs, sugar and vanilla. Add milk and tapioca, stirring constantly.

Pour them into individual cups for custard. Cover each cup firmly with the foil. Pour the water into the pot.

Position the cups on the rack of the pot. Close and secure the lid.

Place the pressure regulator on the vent tube and cook 5 minutes once the pressure regulator begins to rock slowly.

Cool the pot quickly. Let the pudding cool well in the refrigerator.

Nutrition:

Calories: 113

Apple Crisp With Oatmeal

Difficulty Level: 2/5

Preparation time: 5 minutes

Cooking time: 20 minutes

Servings: 4

Ingredients:

4 cups peeled apples and slices

1 tablespoon lemon juice

½ cup quick-cooking oatmeal

¼ cup brown sugar

2 tablespoons flour

1 teaspoon cinnamon

2 tablespoons soft butter

2 cups of water

Directions:

Spray apples with lemon juice. Combine oatmeal, brown sugar, flour and cinnamon.

Cut and add the butter to the oatmeal mixture until a lumpy dough forms. Place the apples in an oiled bowl that fits comfortably in the pot. Spray the oatmeal mixture evenly over apples. Cover the bowl firmly with the foil.

Pour the water into the pot. Position the bowl on the rack of the pot. Close and secure the lid.

Place the pressure regulator on the vent tube and cook 20 minutes once the pressure regulator begins to swing slowly. Cool the pot quickly.

Nutrition:

Calories: 209

Jamaican Cornmeal Porridge

Difficulty Level: 2/5

Preparation time: 5 minutes

Cook time: 16 minutes

Servings: 6

Ingredients:

4 separate cups of water

1 cup of milk

1 cup fine yellow cornmeal

2 cinnamon sticks

3 pepper berries

1 teaspoon vanilla extract

½ teaspoon ground nutmeg

½ cup sweetened condensed milk

Directions:

Add 3 cups of water and 1 cup of milk to the Pressure Pot and stir. In a separate bowl, beat 1 cup of water and cornmeal until completely combined.

Add to the Pressure Pot. Add cinnamon sticks, pepper berries, vanilla extract and nutmeg.

Cover and cook on porridge for 6 minutes. Once the timer is turned off, allow it to release naturally for at least 10 minutes, then quickly release any remaining pressure.

Once done with natural release, open Pressure Pot and beat to remove any lump. Add sweetened condensed milk to sweeten. Enjoy!!

Nutrition:

Calories: 424

Greek Cheesecake with Yogurt

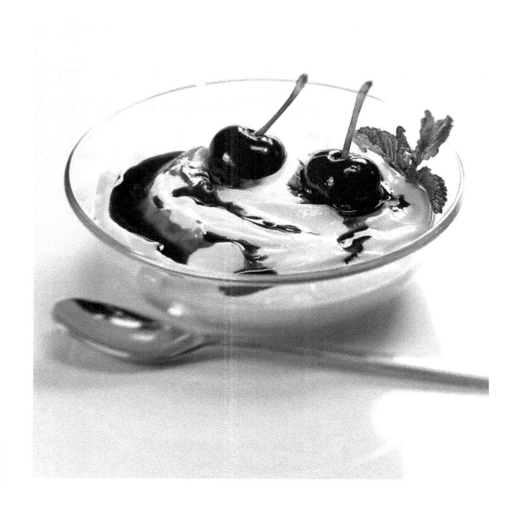

Difficulty Level: 2/5

Preparation time: 20 minutes

Cooking time: 0 minutes

Servings: 12

Ingredients:

1 teaspoon vanilla extract

9 oz. digestive biscuits

3 ½ oz. butter, melted

5 oz. Greek yogurt

16 oz. cream cheese

2 tablespoons honey

4 oz. icing sugar

280 ml double cream

1 cup any jam

Directions:

Add the biscuits to a blender and pulse until crumbled. Transfer the crumbs to a bowl and add the melted butter. Mix well until the crumbs are well coated. Add to the pan and press into the bottom. Refrigerate.

Add Greek yogurt, cream cheese, icing sugar, vanilla, and honey to a bowl. Beat with a mixer until smooth. Add the double cream and beat until well combined.

Add the mixture onto the biscuit crust and top the cheesecake with jam. Refrigerate overnight. Serve.

Nutritional info (per serving):

402 calories;

27 g fat;

36.1 g total carbs;

5.2 g protein

Greek Yogurt and Honey Walnuts
Difficulty Level: 2/5

Preparation time: 5 minutes

Cooking time: 10 minutes

Servings: 6

Ingredients:

- ½ cup honey

- 2 ½ cups strained Greek yogurt

- 1 cup walnuts

- ¾ teaspoon vanilla extract

- Cinnamon powder

Instructions:

Preheat oven to 375 F.

Add the walnuts in a single layer onto the baking sheet. Toast for 8 minutes. Transfer the walnuts to a bowl. Add honey and stir to coat well. Cool down for 2 minutes.

Mix vanilla extract and Greek yogurt and divide among bowls. Add the honey-walnut mixture over the yogurt and add cinnamon powder on top. Serve.

Nutritional info (per serving):

284 calories;

16 g fat;

26.7 g total carbs;

11.8 g protein

Smoked Salmon, Avocado and Cucumber Bites

Difficulty Level: 2/5

Preparation time: 5 minutes

Cooking time: 10 minutes

Servings: 12 bites

Ingredients:

1 large avocado, peeled and pit removed

1 medium cucumber

6 oz. smoked salmon

½ tablespoon lime juice

chives

black pepper

Directions:

Cut the cucumber into ¼ inch thick pieces and lay flat on a plate.

Add the lime juice and the avocado to a bowl and mash with a fork until creamy.

Spread avocado on each cucumber and add a slice of salmon on top.

Add black pepper and chives on each bite.

Once cooked, serve.

Nutritional info (per serving):

46 calories;

3 g fat;

2 g total carbs;

3 g protein

Healthy Coconut Blueberry Balls

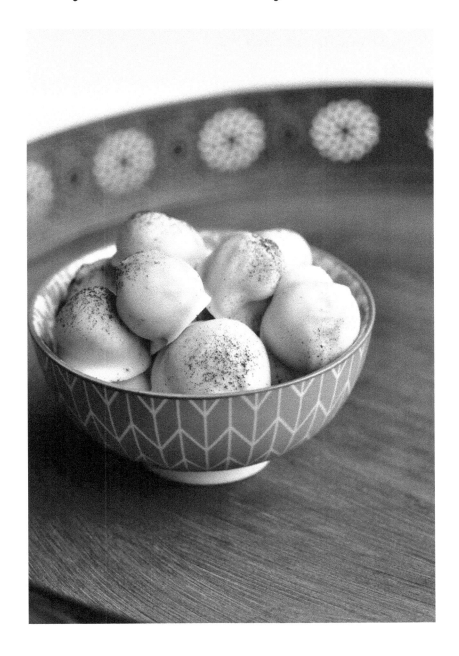

Difficulty Level: 2/5

Preparation Time: 10 minutes

Cooking Time: 10 minutes

Servings: 12

Ingredients:

¼ cup flaked coconut

¼ cup blueberries

½ tsp vanilla

¼ cup honey

½ cup creamy almond butter

¼ tsp cinnamon

1 ½ tbsp chia seeds

¼ cup flaxseed meal

1 cup rolled oats, gluten-free

Directions:

In a large bowl, add oats, cinnamon, chia seeds, and flaxseed meal and mix well.

Add almond butter in microwave-safe bowl and microwave for 30 seconds. Stir until smooth.

Add vanilla and honey in melted almond butter and stir well.

Pour almond butter mixture over oat mixture and stir to combine.

Add coconut and blueberries and stir well.

Make small balls from oat mixture and place onto the baking tray

Serve and enjoy.

Nutritional:

Calories 129,

Fat 7.4g,

Carbohydrates 14.1g,

Sugar 7g,

Protein 4 g,

Cholesterol 0 mg

Roasted Green Beans

Difficulty Level: 2/5

Preparation Time: 10 minutes

Cooking Time: 15 minutes

Servings: 4

Ingredients:

1 lb green beans

4 tbsp parmesan cheese

2 tbsp olive oil

¼ tsp garlic powder

Pinch of salt

Directions:

Preheat the oven to 400 F.

Add green beans in a large bowl.

Add remaining ingredients on top of green beans and toss to coat.

Spread green beans onto the baking tray and roast in preheated oven for 15 minutes. Stir halfway through.

Serve and enjoy.

Nutritional:

Calories 101,

Fat 7.5g,

Carbohydrates 8.3g,

Sugar 1.6g,

Protein 2.6g,

Cholesterol 1mg

Pistachio Balls

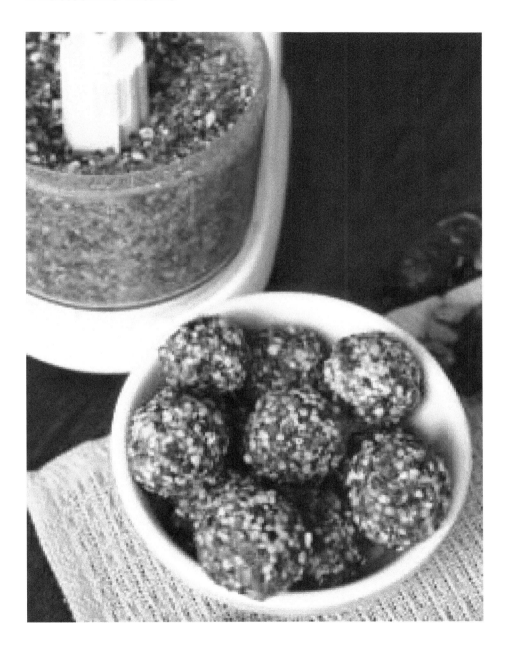

Difficulty Level: 2/5

Preparation Time: 10 minutes

Cooking Time: 5 minutes

Servings: 16

Ingredients:

½ cup pistachios, unsalted

1 cup dates, pitted

½ tsp ground fennel seeds

½ cup raisins

Pinch of pepper

Directions:

Add all ingredients into the food processor and process until well combined.

Make small balls and place onto the baking tray.

Serve and enjoy.

Nutritional:

Calories 55, Fat 0.9g,

Carbohydrates 12.5g,

Sugar 9.9g,

Protein 0.8g,

Cholesterol 0mg

Roasted Almonds

Difficulty Level: 2/5

Preparation Time: 10 minutes

Cooking Time: 20 minutes

Difficulty Level: 2/5: 12

Ingredients:

2 ½ cups almonds

¼ tsp cayenne

¼ tsp ground coriander

¼ tsp cumin

¼ tsp chili powder

1 tbsp fresh rosemary, chopped

1 tbsp olive oil

2 ½ tbsp maple syrup

Pinch of salt

Directions:

Preheat the oven to 325 F.

Spray a baking tray with cooking spray and set aside.

In a mixing bowl, whisk together oil, cayenne, coriander, cumin, chili powder, rosemary, maple syrup, and salt.

Add almond and stir to coat.

Spread almonds onto the prepared baking tray.

Roast almonds in preheated oven for 20 minutes. Stir halfway through.

Serve and enjoy.

Nutritional:

Calories 137,

Fat 11.2g,

Carbohydrates 7.3g,

Sugar 3.3g,

Protein 4.2g,

Cholesterol 0mg

Chocolate Matcha Balls
Difficulty Level: 2/5

Preparation Time: 10 minutes

Cooking Time: 5 minutes

Servings: 15

Ingredients:

2 tbsp unsweetened cocoa powder

3 tbsp oats, gluten-free

½ cup pine nuts

½ cup almonds

1 cup dates, pitted

2 tbsp matcha powder

Directions:

Add oats, pine nuts, almonds, and dates into a food processor and process until well combined.

Place matcha powder in a small dish.

Make small balls from mixture and coat with matcha powder.

Enjoy or store in refrigerator until ready to eat.

Nutritional:

Calories 88,

Fat 4.9g,

Carbohydrates 11.3g,

Sugar 7.8g,

Protein 1.9g,

Cholesterol 0mg

Healthy & Quick Energy Bites
Difficulty Level: 2/5

Preparation Time: 10 minutes

Cooking Time: 0 minutes

Servings: 20

Ingredients:

2 cups cashew nuts

¼ tsp cinnamon

1 tsp lemon zest

4 tbsp dates, chopped

1/3 cup unsweetened shredded coconut

¾ cup dried apricots

Directions:

Line baking tray with parchment paper and set aside.

Add all ingredients in a food processor and process until the mixture is crumbly and well combined.

Make small balls from mixture and place on a prepared baking tray.

Serve and enjoy.

Nutritional:

Calories 100,

Fat 7.5g,

Carbohydrates 7.2g,

Sugar 2.8g,

Protein 2.4g,

Cholesterol omg

Creamy Yogurt Banana Bowls
Difficulty Level: 2/5

Preparation Time: 10 minutes

Cooking Time: 0 minutes

Servings: 4

Ingredients:

2 bananas, sliced

½ tsp ground nutmeg

3 tbsp flaxseed meal

¼ cup creamy peanut butter

4 cups Greek yogurt

Directions:

Divide Greek yogurt between 4 serving bowls and top with sliced bananas.

Add peanut butter in microwave-safe bowl and microwave for 30 seconds.

Drizzle 1 tablespoon of melted peanut butter on each bowl on top of the sliced bananas.

Sprinkle cinnamon and flax meal on top and serve.

Nutritional:

Calories 351,

Fat 13.1g,

Carbohydrates 35.6g,

Sugar 26.1g,

Protein 19.6g,

Cholesterol 15mg

Chocolate Mousse
Difficulty Level: 2/5

Preparation Time: 10 minutes

Cooking Time: 6 minutes

Servings: 5

Ingredients:

4 egg yolks

½ tsp vanilla

½ cup unsweetened almond milk

1 cup whipping cream

¼ cup cocoa powder

¼ cup water

½ cup Swerve

1/8 tsp salt

Directions:

Add egg yolks to a large bowl and whisk until well beaten.

In a saucepan, add swerve, cocoa powder, and water and whisk until well combined.

Add almond milk and cream to the saucepan and whisk until well mix.

Once saucepan mixtures are heated up then turn off the heat.

Add vanilla and salt and stir well.

Add a tablespoon of chocolate mixture into the eggs and whisk until well combined.

Slowly pour remaining chocolate to the eggs and whisk until well combined.

Pour batter into the ramekins.

Pour 1 ½ cups of water into the Pressure Pot then place a trivet in the pot.

Place ramekins on a trivet.

Seal pot with lid and select manual and set timer for 6 minutes.

Release pressure using quick release method than open the lid.

Carefully remove ramekins from the Pressure Pot and let them cool completely.

Serve and enjoy.

Nutrition:

Calories 128,

Fat 11.9g,

Carbohydrates 4g,

Sugar 0.2g,

Protein 3.6g,

Cholesterol 194mg

Carrot Spread
Difficulty Level: 2/5

Preparation time: 10 minutes

Cooking time: 10 minutes

Servings: 4

Ingredients:

¼ cup veggie stock

A pinch of salt and black pepper

1 teaspoon onion powder

½ teaspoon garlic powder

½ teaspoon oregano, dried

1 pound carrots, sliced

½ cup coconut cream

Directions:

In your Pressure Pot, combine all the ingredients except the cream, put the lid on and cook on High for 10 minutes.

Release the pressure naturally for 10 minutes, transfer the carrots mix to food processor, add the cream, pulse well, divide into bowls and serve cold.

Nutrition:

Calories 124,

Fat 1g,

Fiber 2g,

Carbohydrates 5g,

Protein 8g

Decadent Croissant Bread Pudding
Difficulty Level: 2/5

Preparation time: 5 minutes

Cooking time: 15 minutes

Servings: 6

Ingredients

1/2 cup double cream

6 tablespoons honey

1/4 cup rum, divided

2 eggs, whisked

1 teaspoon cinnamon

A pinch of salt

A pinch of grated nutmeg

1 teaspoon vanilla essence

8 croissants, torn into pieces

1 cup pistachios, toasted and chopped

Directions

Spritz a baking pan with cooking spray and set it aside.

In a mixing bowl, whisk the eggs, double cream, honey, rum, cinnamon, salt, nutmeg, and vanilla; whisk until everything is well incorporated.

Place the croissants in the prepared baking dish. Pour the custard over your croissants. Fold in the pistachios and press with a wide spatula.

Add 1 cup of water and metal rack to the inner pot of your Pressure Pot. Lower the baking dish onto the rack.

Secure the lid. Choose the "Manual" mode and cook for 12 minutes at High pressure. Once cooking is complete, use a quick pressure release; carefully remove the lid.

Serve at room temperature or cold. Bon appétit!

Nutrition: (Per serving)

513 Calories;

27.9g Fat;

50.3g Carbohydrates;

12.5g Protein;

25.7g Sugars;

3.8g Fiber

Poached Apples with Greek Yogurt and Granola

Difficulty Level: 2/5

Preparation time: 5 minutes

Cooking time: 15 minutes

Servings 4

Ingredients

4 medium-sized apples, peeled

1/2 cup brown sugar

1 vanilla bean

1 cinnamon stick

1/2 cup cranberry juice

1 cup water

1/2 cup 2% Greek yogurt

1/2 cup granola

Directions

Add the apples, brown sugar, water, cranberry juice, vanilla bean, and cinnamon stick to the inner pot of your Pressure Pot.

Secure the lid. Choose the "Manual" mode and cook for 5 minutes at High pressure. Once cooking is complete, use a natural pressure release for 5 minutes; carefully remove the lid. Reserve poached apples.

Press the "Sauté" button and let the sauce simmer on "Less" mode until it has thickened.

Place the apples in serving bowls. Add the syrup and top each apple with granola and Greek yogurt. Enjoy!

Nutrition: (Per serving)

247 Calories;

3.1g Fat;

52.6g Carbohydrates;

3.5g Protein;

40g Sugars;

5.3g Fiber

Jasmine Rice Pudding with Cranberries
Difficulty Level: 2/5

Preparation time: 5 minutes

Cooking time: 15 minutes

Servings 4

Ingredients

1 cup apple juice

1 heaping tablespoon honey

1/3 cup granulated sugar

1 ½ cups jasmine rice

1 cup water

1/4 teaspoon ground cinnamon

1/4 teaspoon ground cloves

1/3 teaspoon ground cardamom

1 teaspoon vanilla extract

3 eggs, well-beaten

1/2 cup cranberries

Directions

Thoroughly combine the apple juice, honey, sugar, jasmine rice, water, and spices in the inner pot of your Pressure Pot.

Secure the lid. Choose the "Manual" mode and cook for 4 minutes at High pressure. Once cooking is complete, use a natural pressure release for 5 minutes; carefully remove the lid.

Press the "Sauté" button and fold in the eggs. Cook on "Less" mode until heated through.

Ladle into individual bowls and top with dried cranberries. Enjoy!

Nutrition: (Per serving)

402 Calories;

3.6g Fat;

81.1g Carbs;

8.9g Protein;

22.3g Sugars;

2.2g Fiber

Orange and Almond Cupcakes
Difficulty Level: 2/5

Preparation time: 5 minutes

Cooking time: 20 minutes

Servings 9

Ingredients

Cupcakes:

1 orange extract

2 tablespoons olive oil

2 tablespoons ghee, at room temperature

3 eggs, beaten

2 ounces Greek yogurt

2 cups cake flour

A pinch of salt

1 tablespoon grated orange rind

1/2 cup brown sugar

1/2 cup almonds, chopped

Cream Cheese Frosting:

2 ounces cream cheese

1 tablespoon whipping cream

1/2 cup butter, at room temperature

1 ½ cups confectioners' sugar, sifted

1/3 teaspoon vanilla

A pinch of salt

Directions

Mix the orange extract, olive oil, ghee, eggs, and Greek yogurt until well combined.

Thoroughly combine the cake flour, salt, orange rind, and brown sugar in a separate mixing bowl. Add the egg/yogurt mixture to the flour mixture. Stir in the chopped almonds and mix again.

Place parchment baking liners on the bottom of a muffin tin. Pour the batter into the muffin tin.

Place 1 cup of water and metal trivet in the inner pot of your Pressure Pot. Lower the prepared muffin tin onto the trivet.

Secure the lid. Choose the "Manual" mode and cook for 11 minutes at High pressure. Once cooking is complete, use a quick pressure release; carefully remove the lid. Transfer to wire racks.

Meanwhile, make the frosting by mixing all ingredients until creamy. Frost your cupcakes and enjoy!

Nutrition: (Per serving)

392 Calories;

18.7g Fat;

50.1g Carbohydrates;

5.9g Protein;

25.2g Sugars;

0.7g Fiber

Bread Pudding

Difficulty Level: 2/5

Preparation time: 5 minutes

Cooking time: 25 minutes

Servings: 4

Ingredients:

4 egg yolks

3 cups brioche, cubed

2 cups half and half

½ teaspoon vanilla extract

1 cup sugar

2 tablespoons butter, softened

1 cup cranberries

2 cups warm water

½ cup raisins

Zest from 1 lime

Directions:

Grease a baking dish with some butter and set the dish aside. In a bowl, mix the egg yolks with the half and half, cubed brioche, vanilla extract, sugar, cranberries, raisins, and lime zest and stir well. Pour this into greased dish, cover with some aluminum foil and set aside for 10 minutes. Put the dish in the steamer basket of the Pressure Pot, add the warm water to the Pressure Pot, cover, and cook on the Manual setting for 20 minutes. Release the pressure naturally, uncover the Pressure Pot, take the bread pudding out, set it aside to cool down, slice, and serve it.

Nutrition:

Calories: 300

Fat: 7

Fiber: 2

Carbs: 46

Protein: 11

Ruby Pears
Difficulty Level: 2/5

Preparation time: 10 minutes

Cooking time: 10 minutes

Servings: 4

Ingredients:

4 pears

Juice and zest of 1 lemon

26 ounces grape juice

11 ounces currant jelly

4 garlic cloves, peeled

½ vanilla bean

4 peppercorns

2 rosemary sprigs

Directions:

Pour the jelly and grape juice into the Pressure Pot and mix with lemon zest and lemon juice. Dip each pear in this mix, wrap them in aluminum foil and arrange them in the steamer basket of the Pressure Pot. Add the garlic cloves, peppercorns, rosemary, and vanilla bean to the juice mixture, cover the Pressure Pot and cook on the Manual setting for 10 minutes. Release the pressure, uncover the Pressure Pot, take the pears out, unwrap them, arrange them on plates, and serve cold with cooking juice poured on top.

Nutrition:

Calories: 145

Fat: 5.6

Fiber: 6

Carbs: 12

Protein: 12

Lemon Marmalade
Difficulty Level: 2/5

Preparation time: 10 minutes

Cooking time: 15 minutes

Servings: 8

Ingredients:

2 pounds lemons, washed, sliced, and cut into quarters

4 pounds sugar

2 cups water

Directions:

Put the lemon pieces into the Pressure Pot, add the water, cover, and cook on the Manual setting for 10 minutes. Release the pressure naturally, uncover the Pressure Pot, add the sugar, stir, set the Pressure Pot on Manual mode, and cook for 6 minutes, stirring all the time. Divide into jars, and serve when needed.

Nutrition:

Calories: 100

Fat: 2

Fiber: 2

Carbs: 4

Protein: 8

Peach Jam

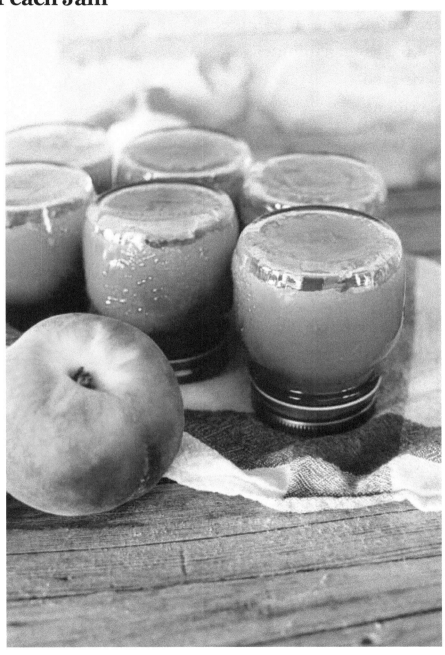

Difficulty Level: 2/5

Preparation time: 10 minutes

Cooking time: 5 minutes

Servings: 6

Ingredients:

4½ cups peaches, peeled and cubed

6 cups sugar

¼ cup crystallized ginger, chopped

1 box fruit pectin

Directions:

Set the Pressure Pot on Manual mode, add the peaches, ginger, and pectin, stir and bring to a boil. Add the sugar, stir, cover and cook on the Manual setting for 5 minutes. Release the pressure, uncover the Pressure Pot, divide the jam into jars, and serve.

Nutrition:

Calories: 50

Fat: 0

Fiber: 1

Carbs: 3

Protein: 0

Sugar: 12

Mango Mug Cake

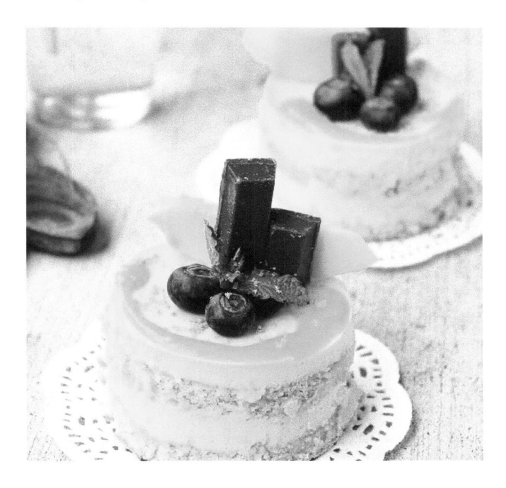

Difficulty Level: 2/5

Preparation time: 5 minutes

Cooking time: 10 minutes

Servings: 2

Ingredients

1 medium-sized mango, peeled and diced

2 eggs

1 teaspoon vanilla

1/4 teaspoon grated nutmeg

1 tablespoon cocoa powder

2 tablespoons honey

1/2 cup coconut flour

Directions:

Combine the coconut flour, eggs, honey, vanilla, nutmeg and cocoa powder in two lightly greased mugs.

Then, add 1 cup of water and a metal trivet to the Pressure Pot. Lower the uncovered mugs onto the trivet.

Secure the lid. Choose the "Manual" mode and High pressure; cook for 10 minutes. Once cooking is complete, use a quick pressure release; carefully remove the lid.

Top with diced mango and serve chilled. Enjoy!

Nutrition:

Calories 268;

Fat 10.5g;

Carbohydrates 34.8g;

Protein 10.6g;

Sugars 31.1g

Chocolate Coffee Pots de Crème

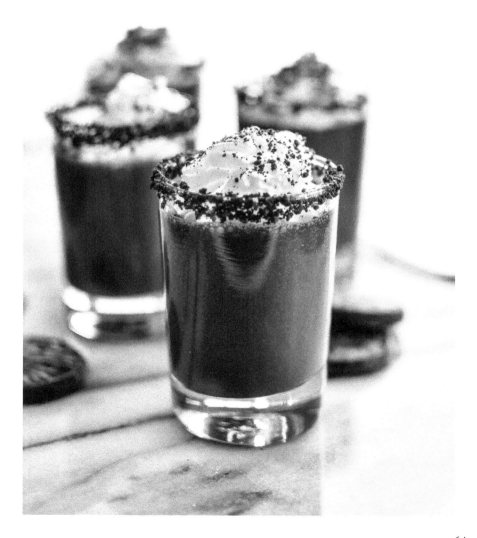

Difficulty Level: 2/5

Preparation time: 10 minutes

Cooking time: 15 minutes

Servings: 6

Ingredients:

1 teaspoon instant coffee

9 ounces chocolate chips

1/2 cup whole milk

1/3 cup sugar

A pinch of pink salt

4 egg yolks

2 cups double cream

Directions:

Place a metal trivet and 1 cup of water in your Pressure Pot.

In a saucepan, bring the cream and milk to a simmer.

Then, thoroughly combine the egg yolks, sugar, instant coffee, and salt. Slowly and gradually whisk in the hot cream mixture.

Whisk in the chocolate chips and blend again. Pour the mixture into mason jars. Lower the jars onto the trivet.

Secure the lid. Choose the "Manual" mode and cook for 6 minutes at High pressure. Once cooking is complete, use a natural pressure release for 10 minutes; carefully remove the lid.

Serve well chilled and enjoy!

Nutrition:

Calories 351;

Fat 19.3g;

Carbohydrates 39.3g;

Protein 5.5g;

Sugars 32.1g

Almond Cherry Crumble Cake

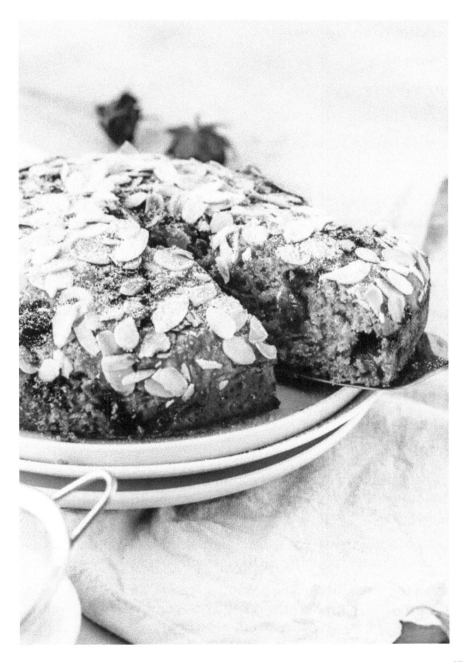

Difficulty Level: 2/5

Preparation time: 5 minutes

Cooking time: 10 minutes

Servings: 4

Ingredients

1/4 cup almonds, slivered

1/2 stick butter, at room temperature

1 teaspoon ground cinnamon

A pinch of grated nutmeg

1 cup rolled oats

1/3 teaspoon ground cardamom

1 teaspoon pure vanilla extract

1/3 cup honey

2 tablespoons all-purpose flour

A pinch of salt

1-pound sweet cherries, pitted

1/3 cup water

Directions

Arrange the cherries on the bottom of the Pressure Pot. Sprinkle cinnamon, cardamom, and vanilla over the top. Add the water and honey.

In a separate mixing bowl, thoroughly combine the butter, oats, and flour. Spread topping mixture evenly over cherry mixture.

Secure the lid. Choose the "Manual" mode and High pressure; cook for 10 minutes. Once cooking is complete, use a natural pressure release; carefully remove the lid.

Serve at room temperature. Bon appétit!

Nutrition:

Calories 335;

Fat 13.4g;

Carbohydrates 60.5g;

Protein 5.9g;

Sugars 38.1g

Orange Butterscotch Pudding

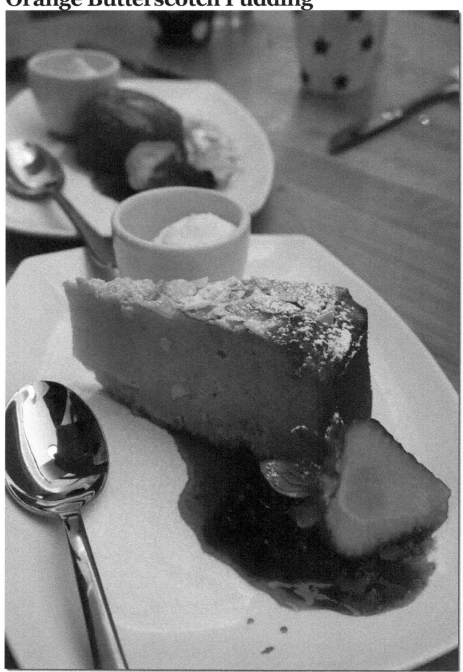

Difficulty Level: 2/5

Preparation time: 10 minutes

Cooking time: 15 minutes

Servings: 4

Ingredients:

4 caramels

2 eggs, well-beaten

1/4 cup freshly squeezed orange juice

1/3 cup sugar

1 cup cake flour

1/2 teaspoon baking powder

1/4 cup milk

1 stick butter, melted

1/2 teaspoon vanilla essence

Sauce:

1/2 cup golden syrup

2 teaspoons corn flour

1 cup boiling water

Directions:

Melt the butter and milk in the microwave. Whisk in the eggs, vanilla, and sugar. After that, stir in the flour, baking powder, and orange juice.

Lastly, add the caramels and stir until everything is well combined and melted.

Divide between the four jars. Add 1 ½ cups of water and a metal trivet to the bottom of the Pressure Pot. Lower the jars onto the trivet.

To make the sauce, whisk the boiling water, corn flour, and golden syrup until everything is well combined. Pour the sauce into each jar.

Secure the lid. Choose the "Steam" mode and cook for 15 minutes under High pressure. Once cooking is complete, use a natural pressure release; carefully remove the lid. Enjoy!

Nutrition:

Calories 565;

Fat 25.9g;

Carbohydrates 79.6g;

Protein 6.4g;

Sugars 51.5g

Recipe for Ruby Pears Delight

Difficulty Level: 2/5

Preparation time: 10 minutes

Cooking time: 10 minutes

Servings: 4

Ingredients:

4 Pears

Grape juice-26 oz.

Currant jelly-11 oz.

4 garlic cloves

Juice and zest of 1 lemon

4 peppercorns

2 rosemary springs

1/2 vanilla bean

Directions:

Pour the jelly and grape juice in your Pressure Pot and mix with lemon zest and juice

In the mix, dip each pear and wrap them in a clean tin foil and place them orderly in the steamer basket of your Pressure Pot

Combine peppercorns, rosemary, garlic cloves and vanilla bean to the juice mixture,

Seal the lid and cook at High for 10 minutes.

Release the pressure quickly, and carefully open the lid; bring out the pears, remove wrappers and arrange them on plates. Serve when cold with toppings of cooking juice.

Nutrition:

Calories: 145

Fat: 5.6

Fiber: 6

Carbs: 12

Protein: 12

Mixed Berry and Orange Compote

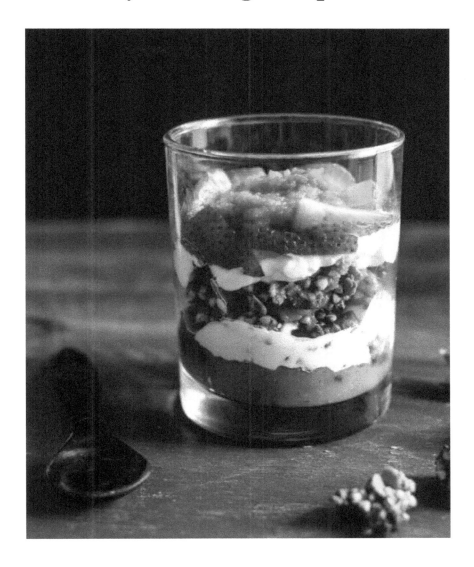

Difficulty Level: 2/5

Preparation time: 15 minutes

Cooking time: 15 minutes

Servings: 4

Ingredients:

1/2-pound strawberries

1 tablespoon orange juice

1/4 teaspoon ground cloves

1/2 cup brown sugar

1 vanilla bean

1-pound blueberries

1/2-pound blackberries

Directions:

Place your berries in the inner pot. Add the sugar and let sit for 15 minutes. Add in the orange juice, ground cloves, and vanilla bean.

Secure the lid. Choose the "Manual" mode and cook for 2 minutes at High pressure. Once cooking is complete, use a natural pressure release for 10 minutes; carefully remove the lid.

As your compote cools, it will thicken. Bon appétit!

Nutrition:

Calories 224;

Fat 0.8g;

Carbohydrates 56.3g;

Protein 2.1g;

Sugars 46.5g

Streuselkuchen with Peaches

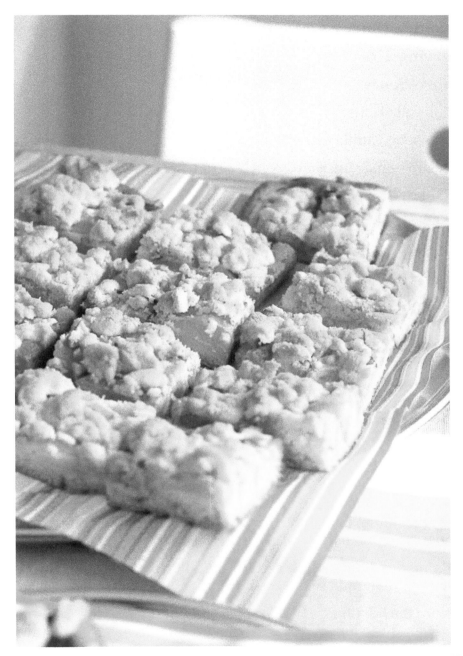

Difficulty Level: 2/5

Preparation time: 10 minutes

Cooking time: 20 minutes

Servings: 6

Ingredients

1 cup rolled oats

1 teaspoon vanilla extract

1/3 cup orange juice

4 tablespoons raisins

2 tablespoons honey

4 tablespoons butter

4 tablespoons all-purpose flour

A pinch of grated nutmeg

1/2 teaspoon ground cardamom

A pinch of salt

1 teaspoon ground cinnamon

6 peaches, pitted and chopped

1/3 cup brown sugar

Directions:

Place the peaches on the bottom of the inner pot. Sprinkle with the cardamom, cinnamon and vanilla. Top with the orange juice, honey, and raisins.

In a mixing bowl, whisk together the butter, oats, flour, brown sugar, nutmeg, and salt. Drop by a spoonful on top of the peaches.

Secure the lid. Choose the "Manual" mode and cook for 8 minutes at High pressure. Once cooking is complete, use a natural pressure release for 10 minutes; carefully remove the lid. Bon appétit!

Nutrition:

329 Calories;

10g Fat;

56g Carbohydrates;

6.9g Protein;

31g Sugars

Fig and Homey Buckwheat Pudding

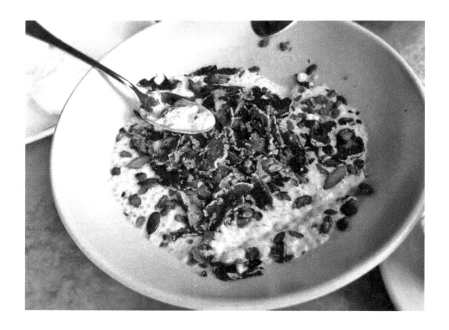

Difficulty Level: 2/5

Preparation time: 10 minutes

Cooking time: 10 minutes

Servings: 4

Ingredients

1/2 teaspoon ground cinnamon

1/2 cup dried figs, chopped

1/3 cup honey

1 teaspoon pure vanilla extract

3 ½ cups milk

1/2 teaspoon pure almond extract

1 ½ cups buckwheat

Directions:

Add all of the above ingredients to your Pressure Pot.

Secure the lid. Choose the "Multigrain" mode and cook for 10 minutes under High pressure. Once cooking is complete, use a natural pressure release; carefully remove the lid.

Serve topped with fresh fruits, nuts or whipped topping. Bon appétit!

Nutrition:

Calories 320;

Fat 7.5g;

Carbohydrates 57.7g;

Protein 9.5g;

Sugars 43.2g

Zingy Blueberry Sauce

Difficulty Level: 2/5

Preparation time: 5 minutes

Cooking time: 20 minutes

Servings: 10

Ingredients

1/4 cup fresh lemon juice

1-pound granulated sugar

1 tablespoon freshly grated lemon zest

1/2 teaspoon vanilla extract

2 pounds fresh blueberries

Directions:

Place the blueberries, sugar, and vanilla in the inner pot of your Pressure Pot.

Secure the lid. Choose the "Manual" mode and cook for 2 minutes at High pressure. Once cooking is complete, use a natural pressure release for 15 minutes; carefully remove the lid.

Stir in the lemon zest and juice. Puree in a food processor; then, strain and push the mixture through a sieve before storing. Enjoy!

Nutrition:

Calories 230;

Fat 0.3g;

Carbohydrates 59g;

Protein 0.7g;

Sugars 53.6g

Chocolate Almond Custard
Difficulty Level: 2/5

Preparation time: 10 minutes

Cooking time: 15 minutes

Servings: 3

Ingredients

3 chocolate cookies, chunks

A pinch of salt

1/4 teaspoon ground cardamom

3 tablespoons honey

1/4 teaspoon freshly grated nutmeg

2 tablespoons butter

3 tablespoons whole milk

1 cup almond flour

3 eggs

1 teaspoon pure vanilla extract

Directions:

In a mixing bowl, beat the eggs with butter. Now, add the milk and continue mixing until well combined.

Add the remaining ingredients in the order listed above. Divide the batter among 3 ramekins.

Add 1 cup of water and a metal trivet to the Pressure Pot. Cover ramekins with foil and lower them onto the trivet.

Secure the lid and select "Manual" mode. Cook at High pressure for 12 minutes. Once cooking is complete, use a quick release; carefully remove the lid.

Transfer the ramekins to a wire rack and allow them to cool slightly before serving. Enjoy!

Nutrition:

Calories 304;

Fat 18.9g;

Carbohydrates 23.8g;

Protein 10g;

Sugars 21.1g

Honey Stewed Apples

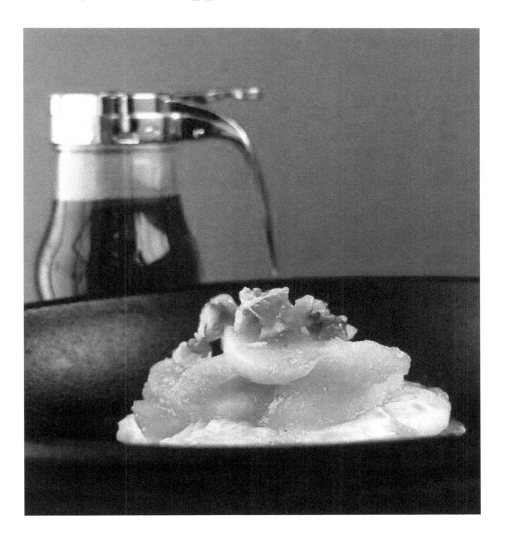

Difficulty Level: 2/5

Preparation time: 5 minutes

Cooking time: 5 minutes

Servings: 4

Ingredients

2 tablespoons honey

1 teaspoon ground cinnamon

1/2 teaspoon ground cloves

4 apples

Directions

Add all ingredients to the inner pot. Now, pour in 1/3 cup of water.

Secure the lid. Choose the "Manual" mode and cook for 2 minutes at High pressure. Once cooking is complete, use a quick pressure release; carefully remove the lid.

Serve in individual bowls. Bon appétit!

Nutrition:

Calories 128;

Fat 0.3g;

Carbohydrates 34.3g;

Protein 0.5g;

Sugars 27.5g

Greek-Style Compote with Yogurt

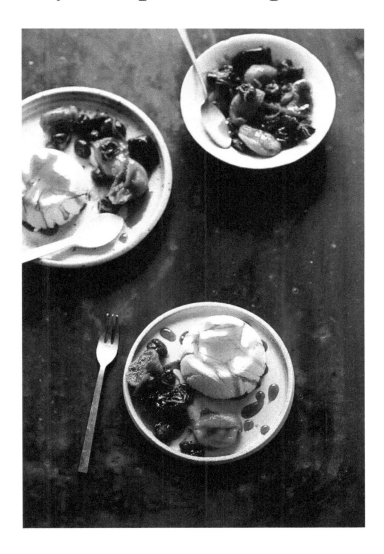

Difficulty Level: 2/5

Preparation time: 5 minutes

Cooking time: 15 minutes

Servings: 4

Ingredients:

1 cup Greek yoghurt

1 cup pears

4 tablespoons honey

1 cup apples

1 vanilla bean

1 cinnamon stick

1/2 cup caster sugar

1 cup rhubarb

1 teaspoon ground ginger

1 cup plums

Directions:

Place the fruits, ginger, vanilla, cinnamon, and caster sugar in the inner pot of your Pressure Pot.

Secure the lid. Choose the "Manual" mode and cook for 2 minutes at High pressure. Once cooking is complete, use a natural pressure release for 10 minutes; carefully remove the lid.

Meanwhile, whisk the yogurt with the honey.

Serve your compote in individual bowls with a dollop of honeyed Greek yogurt. Enjoy!

Nutrition:

Calories 304;

Fat 0.3g;

Carbohydrates 75.4g;

Protein 5.1g;

Sugars 69.2g

Butterscotch Lava Cakes
Difficulty Level: 2/5

Preparation time: 5 minutes

Cooking time: 15 minutes

Servings: 6

Ingredients

7 tablespoons all-purpose flour

A pinch of coarse salt

6 ounces butterscotch morsels

3/4 cup powdered sugar

1/2 teaspoon vanilla extract

3 eggs, whisked

1 stick butter

Directions

Add 1 ½ cups of water and a metal rack to the Pressure Pot. Line a standard-size muffin tin with muffin papers.

In a microwave-safe bowl, microwave butter and butterscotch morsels for about 40 seconds. Stir in the powdered sugar.

Add the remaining ingredients Spoon the batter into the prepared muffin tin.

Secure the lid. Choose the "Manual" and cook at High pressure for 10 minutes. Once cooking is complete, use a quick release; carefully remove the lid.

To remove, let it cool for 5 to 6 minutes. Run a small knife around the sides of each cake and serve. Enjoy!

Nutrition:

Calories 393;

Fat 21.1g;

Carbohydrates 45.6g;

Protein 5.6g;

Sugars 35.4g

Vanilla Bread Pudding with Apricots

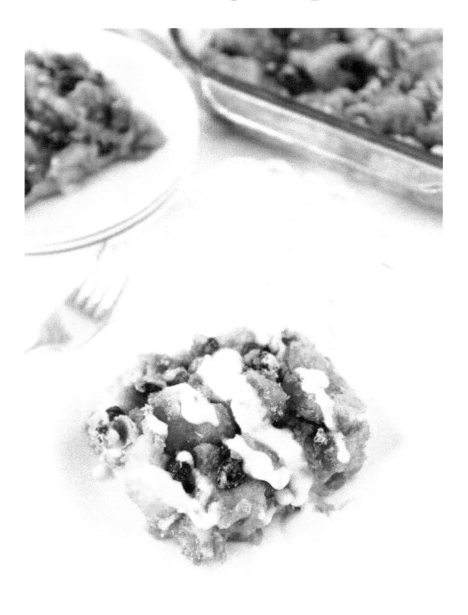

Difficulty Level: 2/5

Preparation time: 5 minutes

Cooking time: 15 minutes

Servings: 6

Ingredients

2 tablespoons coconut oil

1 1/3 cups heavy cream

4 eggs, whisked

1/2 cup dried apricots, soaked and chopped

1 teaspoon cinnamon, ground

1/2 teaspoon star anise, ground

A pinch of grated nutmeg

A pinch of salt

1/2 cup granulated sugar

2 tablespoons molasses

2 cups milk

4 cups Italian bread, cubed

1 teaspoon vanilla paste

Directions

Add 1 ½ cups of water and a metal rack to the Pressure Pot.

Grease a baking dish with a nonstick cooking spray. Throw the bread cubes into the prepared baking dish.

In a mixing bowl, thoroughly combine the remaining ingredients Pour the mixture over the bread cubes. Cover with a piece of foil, making a foil sling.

Secure the lid. Choose the "Porridge" mode and High pressure; cook for 15 minutes. Once cooking is complete, use a quick pressure release; carefully remove the lid. Enjoy!

Nutrition:

Calories 410;

Fat 24.3g;

Carbohydrates 37.4g;

Protein 11.5g;

Sugars 25.6g

Mediterranean-Style Carrot Pudding
Difficulty Level: 2/5

Preparation time: 15 minutes

Cooking time: 15 minutes

Servings: 4

Ingredients

1/3 cup almonds, ground

1/4 cup dried figs, chopped

2 large-sized carrots, shredded

1/2 cup water

1 ½ cups milk

1/2 teaspoon ground star anise

1/3 teaspoon ground cardamom

1/4 teaspoon kosher salt

1/3 cup granulated sugar

2 eggs, beaten

1/2 teaspoon pure almond extract

1/2 teaspoon vanilla extract

1 ½ cups jasmine rice

Directions

Place the jasmine rice, milk, water, carrots, and salt in your Pressure Pot.

Stir to combine and secure the lid. Choose "Manual" and cook at High pressure for 10 minutes. Once cooking is complete, use a natural release for 15 minutes; carefully remove the lid.

Now, press the "Sauté" button and add the sugar, eggs, and almonds; stir to combine well. Bring to a boil; press the "Keep Warm/Cancel" button.

Add the remaining ingredients and stir; the pudding will thicken as it sits. Bon appétit!

Nutrition:

331 Calories;

17.2g Fat;

44.5g Carbohydrates;

13.9g Protein;

19.5g Sugars

Oatmeal Cakes With Mango

Difficulty Level: 2/5

Preparation time: 5 minutes

Cooking time: 17 minutes

Servings: 2

Ingredients:

Hot cakes:

2 cups of oatmeal

3 eggs

1 tablespoon baking powder

1¼ cups of natural yogurt

1 teaspoon vanilla extract

1 cup chopped apple in small cubes

Oil spray

Mango honey (syrup):

2 cups diced mango

Orange juice

1 tablespoon maple honey

1 tablespoon vanilla extract

1 cinnamon stick

Directions:

In the pot, place all the ingredients of mango honey. Cover with valve open and cook at medium-high temperature until it whistles (in about 5 minutes). Reduce the temperature to low, remove the lid and continue cooking for 4 more minutes. Let cool a little and blend for a few seconds until you get a homogeneous mixture.

Also, blend all the ingredients of the hotcakes (except apple and oil spray) at speed 6, for 1 minute (until you get a homogeneous consistency). Pour into the Mixing Bowl and stir with the apple pieces, using the Balloon Whisk.

Preheat at medium-high temperature for 2 minutes. Reduce the temperature to low and sprinkle some oil spray.

Cook 6 to 8 hotcakes, for 2 minutes per side. Repeat with the remaining mixture.

Nutrition:

Calories: 245

Carbohydrates: 51.6g

Fat: 4.3g

Protein: 8.4g

Sugar: 8g

Cholesterol: 2mg

Wrapped Eggs
Difficulty Level: 2/5

Preparation time: 5 minutes

Cooking time: 17 minutes

Servings: 6

Ingredients:

6 cooked eggs, without shell

1 uncooked egg

1 pound (½ kg) ground turkey meat low fat

¼ cup finely chopped onion

¼ cup finely chopped jalapeños

¼ cup of ground bread

Mustard Dressing:

½ cup chicken broth

½ cup double cream (heavy cream)

1 teaspoon Dijon mustard

1 teaspoon tarragon leaves

1 teaspoon fine cornmeal (cornstarch) —optional

Directions:

In the pot, mix the chicken broth, double cream, mustard and tarragon leaves. Cook at medium-high temperature until the dressing begins to thicken, in about 8 minutes. Stir occasionally. If you want the sauce to be thicker, you can add 1 teaspoon of fine cornmeal, and beat well until all the lumps are dissolved.

In a bowl, combine turkey, onion, jalapenos and raw egg. Add the breadcrumbs, and season with salt and pepper to taste.

Make 6 thin burgers with the meat mixture and use them to wrap the cooked eggs.

Preheat a skillet at medium-high temperature for about 3 minutes or until, after spraying a few drops of water, they roll on the surface without evaporating. Immediately reduce the temperature to medium, and cook the wrapped eggs for 4 minutes, with the lid ajar.

Turn and cook for 5 more minutes with the lid closed. Make sure the meat is fully cooked before removing the eggs from the stove. Serve with the dressing.

Nutrition:

Calories:150

Carbohydrates: 21g

Fat: 7g

Protein: 2g

Sugar: 20g

Cholesterol: 5mg

Zucchini Chips

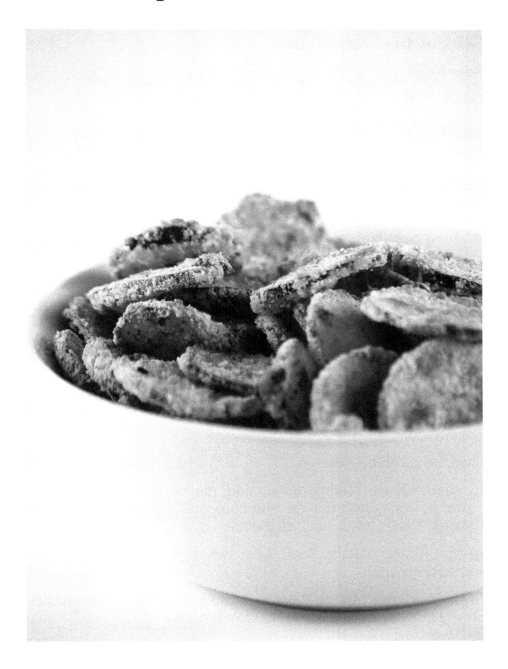

Difficulty Level: 2/5

Preparation time: 5 minutes

Cooking time: 15 minutes

Servings: 4

Ingredients:

1 pound (½ kg) zucchini, sliced

1 cup mayonnaise

½ cup sour cream

1 tablespoon sriracha sauce (or hot chili sauce), or to taste

2 tablespoons honey

½ cup chives (scallion/green onion), chopped

½ cup of breadcrumbs

½ cup parmesan cheese

1 teaspoon red paprika (paprika)

2 eggs

1 teaspoon of water

Directions:

Slice the zucchini. Reserve.

In the 2-Quart Mixing Bowl, add mayonnaise, sour cream, sriracha, honey and chives. Combine well with the help of the Balloon Whisk, cover and refrigerate.

In the 3-quart Mixing Bowl, beat the eggs with a teaspoon of water; reservation.

In the 1-quarter Mixing Bowl, mix the ground bread, Parmesan cheese and paprika. Reserve separately.

Dip the zucchini slices in the beaten egg, then cover them with the ground bread mixture. Place each slice in the Cookie Tray.

Preheat the oven to 400 F / 204 C. Place the tray inside the oven and cook for 8 minutes. Flip the chips with the help of the Spatula and bake for 7 more minutes.

Serve with the honey and sriracha sauce. Bon Appetite!

Nutrition:

Calories: 344

Carbohydrates: 46g

Fat: 9.3g

Protein: 18g

Sugar: 4.8g

Cholesterol: 0mg

Rice Pudding
Difficulty Level: 2/5

Preparation time: 5 minutes

Cooking time: 10 minutes

Servings: 10

Ingredients:

6 cups of white rice, previously cooked

2 cups of double cream (heavy whipping cream)

1 cup coconut milk

3 cups of skim milk

2 cinnamon sticks (cinnamon stick)

1 teaspoon allspice

1 teaspoon nutmeg

½ cup brown sugar

Cinnamon powder to taste

Directions:

In the pot, add all the ingredients.

Cook at medium-high temperature for 10 minutes; Stir frequently.

Garnish with a pinch of cinnamon.

Nutrition:

Calories: 344

Carbohydrates: 46g

Fat: 9.3g

Protein: 18g

Sugar: 4.8g

Cholesterol: 0mg

Grilled Pineapple Sandwich

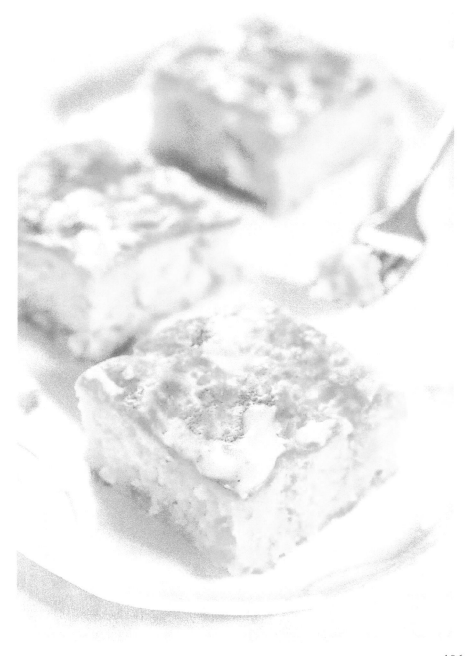

Difficulty Level: 2/5

Preparation time: 10 minutes

Cooking time: 7 minutes

Servings: 4

Ingredients:

8 slices of pineapple

½ cup macadamia nuts, chopped

½ cup chocolate cream and hazelnut spread

¼ cup double cream

½ cup mascarpone Italian cheese

1 teaspoon whipped cream

4 cherries

Directions:

Preheat the skillet at medium temperature for 3 minutes. Add the macadamia nuts and store them for 3 minutes, stir constantly.

Preheat the Round Grill at medium-high temperature for 3 minutes. Add the pineapple slices and roast each side for 2 minutes.

In a bowl, add the chocolate cream, double cream and mascarpone cheese; stir until a uniform mixture is achieved. Spread four slices of pineapple with the mixture and cover with the remaining slices to form the sandwiches. Garnish with the cream, cherries and nuts.

Nutrition:

Calories: 344

Carbohydrates: 46g

Fat: 9.3g

Protein: 18g

Sugar: 4.8g

Cholesterol: 0mg

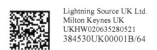

Lightning Source UK Ltd.
Milton Keynes UK
UKHW020635280521
384530UK00001B/64